I0466089

UNDERSTANDING AVIAN INFLUENZA

Unraveling the Bird Flu Mystery.

Amelia R. Morris

Copyright Page

Copyright © (Amelia R. Morris), (2024).

All rights reserved. No part of this publication may be reproduced, distributed, or transmitted in any form or by any means, including photocopying, recording, or other electronic or mechanical methods, without the prior written permission of the publisher, except in the case of brief quotations embodied in critical reviews and certain other noncommercial uses permitted by copyright law.

Table Of Contents

INTRODUCTION TO AVIAN INFLUENZA

Virus Origins

Avian influenza, commonly referred to as "bird flu," is a viral illness primarily impacting birds but with the potential for sporadic transmission to humans. In humans, the predominant strain is Influenza A(H5N1), which can result in severe respiratory complications. Individuals in frequent contact with poultry, waterfowl (such as ducks and geese), and livestock are at heightened risk of contracting the virus.

The emergence of the novel influenza A(H7N9) virus marked a significant milestone, representing the first instance of a low-pathogenic avian influenza virus (LPAI) causing severe illness in humans and eventually evolving into a highly pathogenic form. Avian influenza strains are classified as either "low-pathogenic" or "highly pathogenic" based on their capacity to induce severe illness and mortality in poultry, as well as their possession of specific genetic markers.

Research incorporating active surveillance, analysis of historical virus data, and evolutionary studies has suggested that A(H7) viruses likely originated from domestic ducks before transferring to chickens in China. Subsequently, genetic reassortment with poultry influenza A(H9N2) contributed to the emergence of the A(H7N9) strain capable of infecting humans. Although the precise reservoir for this novel virus remains unidentified, continuous circulation of various A(H9N2) genotypes in farmed poultry may have facilitated antigenic changes and adaptation over time.

Experimental evidence indicates that the susceptibility, transmission, and viral shedding of A(H7N9) in birds are influenced by the species involved. Since its appearance in 2013, the evolution of A(H7N9) viruses within poultry populations has led to genetic diversity across different regions in China, culminating in the emergence of a highly pathogenic variant.

The genetic makeup of the A(H7N9) virus raises concerns regarding its pandemic potential, including its ability to bind to receptors present in both human and avian influenza viruses, thereby impacting its potential for sustained human-to-human transmission and replication.

While A(H7N9) has not been detected in Europe, its initial identification in China in March 2013 prompted concern. The majority of human cases were reported in Mainland China between 2013 and 2017, with chickens being the primary poultry species affected. The mutation of the low-pathogenic A(H7N9) virus into a highly pathogenic form occurred in late 2016, with human infections linked to direct contact with birds or visits to live bird markets.

Following the implementation of a large-scale vaccination program against A(H7N9) in poultry in China, there has been a significant decrease in outbreaks and human cases. Since 2018, only sporadic human cases have been reported. The clinical presentation of A(H7N9) infection varies from mild to severe, with a notable proportion of patients requiring hospitalization, particularly among older males. The outbreak demonstrates a seasonal pattern, peaking between November and March, with sporadic cases during the summer months. Although small family clusters have been reported, sustained person-to-person transmission has not been definitively established.

Global Impact

Avian flu infections (AIVs) are around the world testing because of far reaching course and high death rates. Exceptionally pathogenic avian flu (HPAI) strains like H5N1 have caused critical episodes in birds. Starting around 2003 to 14 July 2023, the World Wellbeing Association (WHO) has archived 878 instances of HPAI H5N1 disease in people and 458 (52.16%) fatalities in 23 nations. Ongoing flare-ups in wild birds, homegrown birds, ocean lions, minks, and so forth, and the event of hereditary varieties among HPAI H5N1 strains raise worries about possible transmission and general wellbeing gambles.

The world is faced by numerous significant public health challenges, some of which comprise possibly devastating global dangers. Prime among these is the danger of a flu pandemic. It is plausible made all the more genuine by the emergenceand multi-local spread of profoundly pathogenic avian influenza A (H5N1). This epizootic has caught the attention of the global local area and cautioned the world to the possibilities of a possibly crushing human health challenge. Since its first appearance in quite a while in1997

the H5N1 infection has not disappeared, nor has it

turn out to be less deadly nor less boundless in birds. On the contrary, its advancing environment and determination in wild creature supplies addresses a genuine and supported hazard,increasing the likelihood that it might transform into a pandemic strain. However long this infection keeps on coursing in animals, the gamble of a flu pandemic is immediately present.

Flu pandemics are natural phenomena that have happened intermittently for quite a long time.

Further, the circumstances for the rise and spread of novel flu infections have not subsided.

The geographic tirelessness of H5N1, its advanced spread and wide host range is both exceptional and worrisome. Never before has an exceptionally pathogenic avian influenza caused episodes in such countless nations at once;never before has the illness spread so broadly and rapidly to influence such enormous topographical regions. The H5N1 epizootic is the most apparent and troubling danger by and by. The Possibility, nonetheless, of other pandemic specialists arising should not be ignored.

EPIDEMIOLOGY AND TRANSMISSION

Spread Among Birds

Avian (bird) flu (influenza) infections generally don't infect individuals(people), there have been a few uncommon instances of human disease with these infections. Ailment in people from avian flu infection contaminations have gone in seriousness from no side effects or gentle sickness to extreme illness that brought about death. Avian flu A(H7N9) infection and profoundly pathogenic avian flu (HPAI) A(H5N1) and A(H5N6) infections have been answerable for most human sickness from avian flu infections detailed overall to date, including the most difficult ailments with high mortality.

Contaminated birds shed avian flu infections through their spit, mucous and defecation. Different creatures tainted with avian flu infections might have infection present in respiratory emissions, various organs, blood, or in other body liquids, including creature milk. Human diseases with avian flu infections can happen when infection gets into an individual's eyes, nose or mouth, or is breathed in. This can happen when infection is in the air (in drops, little spray particles, or conceivably residue) and stores on the bodily fluid films of the eyes or an individual inhales it in, or potentially when an individual contacts something tainted by infections and afterward contacts their mouth, eyes or nose.

Avian flu infections have been identified in numerous different species. Keep away from contact with surfaces that seem, by all accounts, to be defiled with creature dung, crude milk, litter, or materials tainted by birds or different creatures with thought or affirmed avian flu infection disease. CDC has data about insurances to take with wild birds, poultry and different creatures.

CDC has direction for explicit gatherings with openness to poultry and other possibly contaminated creatures, including poultry or dairy laborers, for instance, and individuals answering bird influenza flare-ups.

Human Infection Risks

The gamble of contamination is low for the overall population who have restricted contact with tainted creatures; those with close contact to contaminated creatures are at expanded risk, and ought to play it safe.

Human disease with avian flu A(H5N1) is interesting.

Beginning around 1997, there have been more than 900 human instances of avian flu A(H5N1) announced around the world, generally happening in Africa and Asia. The quantity of human cases has diminished considerably starting around 2015. This reduction might be credited to the utilization of poultry immunizations, avoidance and control drives, and possibly changes in the infection.

The transcendent avian flu A(H5N1) infections presently coursing around the world among birds and different creatures are unique in relation to prior A(H5N1) infections. Avian flu infections constantly change, which can influence how effectively the infection spreads from birds to different creatures, including people, and furthermore the way that serious ailment is.

While by and large, the gamble of disease was most elevated for those venturing out to regions in Asia and Africa, avian flu A(H5N1) has as of late spread all through Europe and North America and has been distinguished in Focal and South America, and Antarctica. In 2022, the infection became boundless across Canada through the movement of wild birds, and has impacted numerous poultry ranches and a wide range of types of wild birds and other natural life. Most as of late, A(H5N1) has additionally been identified in animals, like dairy steers and goats.

Barely any human cases related with the 2021-2024 avian flu A(H5N1) episode have been recognized. The quantity of A(H5N1) human cases revealed overall is followed and announced in the Human Arising Respiratory Microorganism Release.

There has just been one human instance of A(H5N1) at any point detailed in Canada. A Canadian occupant passed on from avian flu A(H5N1) in mid 2014 subsequent to getting back from an outing to China, where they were reasonably tainted.

Avian flu isn't known to be a sanitation concern. There is no proof that eating completely cooked business poultry, eggs and meat could communicate avian flu to people. Endlessly milk items that are purified are likewise protected to drink.

Safe food taking care of practices ought to be followed.

Such practices incorporate handwashing and keeping poultry, meat, eggs and egg items separate from other food items to stay away from cross tainting.

Sanitization of milk is a prerequisite available to be purchased of cow's milk in Canada.

Sanitization guarantees the milk we drink is protected by killing harmful microorganisms and infections while holding the dietary properties of milk.

AVIAN INFLUENZA VIRUS: TYPES

Classification

There are four kinds of flu (seasonal) infections: A, B, C and D. Wild sea-going birds, including gulls, terns, and shorebirds, and wild waterfowl, for example, ducks, geese and swans are viewed as repositories (has) for avian flu And infections.

Subtypes of Flu And Infections

Flu And infections are isolated into subtypes based on two proteins on the outer layer of the infection: hemagglutinin (HA) and neuraminidase (NA). There are 18 known HA subtypes and 11 known NA subtypes. In birds, 16 HA and 9 NA subtypes have been distinguished. (Two extra subtypes, H17N10 and H18N11, have been distinguished in bats.) Various blends of HA and NA proteins are conceivable. For instance, an "A(H7N2) infection" assigns a flu An infection subtype that has a HA 7 protein and a NA 2 protein. Likewise, an "A(H5N1)" infection has a HA 5 protein and a NA 1 protein.

All known subtypes of flu And infections can contaminate birds, with the exception of subtypes A(H17N10) and A(H18N11), which have just been viewed as in bats. Just two flu An infection subtypes A(H1N1)pdm09, and A(H3N2), are right now coursing among individuals. Flu And infections have been identified and are known to course in seven different creature species or gatherings, including people, wild water birds, homegrown poultry, pig, ponies, canines and bats. In numerous other creature species, avian flu And infections have been accounted for to cause periodic diseases, however don't consistently spread among them (e.g., felines and seals). Equine (horse) flu A(H3N8) infection regularly courses and can cause sickness in ponies, and canine (canine) flu A(H3N2) infection regularly circles and can cause disease in canines.

There are four types of influenza (occasional) contaminations: A, B, C and D. Wild maritime birds, including gulls, terns, and shorebirds, and wild waterfowl, for instance, ducks, geese and swans are seen as stores (has) for avian influenza A diseases.

Subtypes of Influenza A Contaminations

Influenza A contaminations are disconnected into subtypes in light of two proteins on the external layer of the disease: hemagglutinin (HA) and neuraminidase (NA). There are 18 known HA subtypes and 11 known NA subtypes. In birds, 16 HA and 9 NA subtypes have been recognized. (An additional two subtypes, H17N10 and H18N11, have been recognized in bats.) Different mixes of HA and NA proteins are possible. For example, an "A(H7N2) disease" relegates an influenza A contamination subtype that has a HA 7 protein and a NA 2 protein. Moreover, an "A(H5N1)" disease has a HA 5 protein and a NA 1 protein.

All known subtypes of influenza A diseases can pollute birds, except for subtypes A(H17N10) and A(H18N11), which have recently been considered to be in bats. Only two influenza A contamination subtypes A(H1N1)pdm09, and A(H3N2), are correct now flowing among people. Influenza A diseases have been recognized and are known to occur in seven different animal species or social occasions, including individuals, wild water birds, local poultry, pigs, horses, canines and bats. In various other animal species, avian influenza A contaminations have been represented to cause occasional sicknesses, but don't predictably spread among them (e.g., cats and seals). Equine (horse) influenza A(H3N8) contamination consistently courses and can cause ailment in horses, and canine (canine) influenza A(H3N2) contamination routinely circles and can cause sickness in poultry (canine).

Genetic Variation

Avian flu infection H9N2 has turned into the prevailing subtype of flu which is endemic in poultry. The hemagglutinin, one of eight protein-coding qualities, assumes a significant part during the beginning phase of contamination. The versatile advancement and the emphatically chosen locales of the HA (the glycoprotein atom) of H9N2 subtype infections were examined. Exploring 68 hemagglutinin H9N2 avian flu infection segregates in China and phylogenetic examination, it was fundamental that these disengages were circulated topographically from 1994, and were completely gotten from the Eurasian genealogy. H9N2 avian flu infection disengages from homegrown poultry in China were particularly phylogenetically from those separated in Hong Kong, including infections which had contaminated people. Seven amino corrosive replacements (2T, 3T, 14T, 165D, 197A, 233Q, 380R) were distinguished in the HA potentially because of positive determination pressure. Aside from the 380R site, the other emphatically chosen destinations distinguished were totally situated close to the receptor-restricting site of the HA1 strain. In light of epidemiological and phylogenetics examination, the H9N2 plague in China was separated into three gatherings: the 1994-1997 gathering, the 1998-1999 gathering, and the 2000-2007 gathering. By examining these three gatherings utilizing the most extreme probability assessment strategy, there were more specific destinations in the 1994-1997 and 1998-1999 scourge bunch than the 2000-2007 gatherings. This demonstrates that those identified chosen destinations are changed during various pandemic periods and the advancement of H9N2 is presently sluggish. The antigenic determinant or other key utilitarian amino corrosive destinations ought to be of concern on the grounds that their nearby locales have been feeling the squeeze. The outcomes give additional proof that the pathogenic changes in the H9N2 subtype are expected predominantly to re-combination with other profoundly pathogenic avian flu infections.

CLINICAL SIGNS AND DIAGNOSIS

Avian Symptoms

Bird influenza, likewise called avian flu, is a viral contamination that can taint birds, yet additionally people and different creatures. Most types of the infection are limited to birds.

H5N1 is the most well-known type of bird influenza. It's destructive to birds and can undoubtedly influence people and different creatures that interact with a transporter. As per the World Wellbeing OrganizationTrusted Source, H5N1 was first found in quite a while in 1997 and has killed almost 60 percentTrusted Wellspring of those tainted.

Presently, the infection isn't known to spread through human-to-human contact. In any case, a few specialists stress that

H5N1 might represent a gamble of turning into a pandemic danger to people.

Signs of less severe highly pathogenic avian influenza:

- Depression
- Reduced food intake
- Weakness
- Soft-shelled eggs
- Reduced egg laying
- Dark, thickened or drooping combs and wattles
- Diarrhoea
- Coughing
- Difficulty breathing
- Increased deaths.

Signs of low pathogenic avian influenza: depression

- Reduced food intake
- Reduced laying
- Nasal discharge, coughing, sneezing diarrhoea
- Increased deaths.

Assuming you're presented to bird influenza, you ought to tell staff before you show up at the specialist's office or medical clinic. Cautioning them quite a bit early will permit them to play it safe to safeguard staff and different patients prior to really focusing on you.

Diagnostic Techniques

Individuals in the EU giving serious intense respiratory contaminations (SARI) or flu like diseases (ILI) and a background marked by openness to dead or debilitated poultry, wild birds or different warm blooded creatures probably tainted with A(H5N1) avian flu infections will require cautious examination, the board and contamination control. Neurological side effects have additionally been seen in vertebrates tainted with avian flu infections. Assuming transmission to people happen, other non-respiratory side effects could perhaps at the same time happen.

Clinicians ought to consider testing seriously sick patients for flu, who present with respiratory and furthermore different side effects (for example neurological). Proper examples for flu tests ought to be quickly taken and handled from patients with pertinent openness history inside 10-14 days going before the side effect beginning. On the off chance that positive examples can't be subtyped, they ought to be imparted to the public reference lab of the particular country (Public Flu Habitats - NICs(link is outside)).

With routine symptomatic research facility tests for occasional flu infections, human contamination with A(H5Nx) infections ought to be positive for flu An infection, and negative for flu B, A(H1), A(H1)pdm09 and A(H3) infections. Such non-occasional flu type An infection separates, or clinical examples that can't be subtyped, ought to be shipped off the individual NIC. On the off chance that they are affirmed positive for H5 infection, the examples ought to be sent further along to a WHO Teaming up Community for Reference and Exploration on Flu (WHO-CCRRI).

The affirmation of a useful avian flu disease in an individual (suggestive or asymptomatic) with a positive PCR ought to incorporate continued testing to bar a bogus positive sign. Genuine up-sides ought to be exposed to resulting infection sequencing to deliver full-length genomes for additional investigation and infection development. Examples ought to be imparted to reference research centers and WHO-CCRRIs for infection characterisation as illustrated in the ECDC direction report.

Serological examinations are likewise expected to distinguish seroconversion for case ascertainment. Be that as it may, for some infection energy discoveries, it very well may be trying to affirm or preclude a genuine disease. More work should be performed all around the world to foster standards on the most proficient method to arrange such uncertain outcomes.

Reference infections and sera against reference infections should be grown, continually refreshed, and gave to nations to research transmission occasions and affirm contaminations serologically. This is additionally expected to help risk appraisals and lead bigger examinations in populace gatherings (like poultry laborers, cullers, slaughterhouse laborers) at high gamble of openness to avian flu infections or to possibly tainted birds.

ZOONOTIC POTENTIAL

Transmission Dynamics

Openness to contaminated poultry is an associated cause with avian flu (H5N1) infection diseases in people. We identified irresistible beads and vapor sprayers during research facility reproduced handling of asymptomatic chickens contaminated with human-(clades 1 and 2.2.1) and avian-(clades 1.1, 2.2, and 2.1) beginning H5N1 infections.

We identified less airborne irresistible particles in recreated handling of contaminated ducks. Flu infection credulous chickens and ferrets presented to the air space in which infected chickens were handled became contaminated and kicked the bucket, recommending that the butcher of contaminated chickens is a productive wellspring of airborne infection that can contaminate birds and vertebrates. We didn't identify reliable diseases in ducks and ferrets presented to the air space in which infection tainted ducks were handled. Our outcomes support the speculation that airborne transmission of HPAI infections can happen among poultry and from poultry to people during home or live-poultry market butcher of contaminated poultry.

Watchwords: H5N1 exceptionally pathogenic avian flu, poultry, airborne transmission, spray, bead, infections
Beginning around 2003, roughly 850 human instances of Eurasian A/goose/Guangdong/1/1996 (Gs/GD) heredity H5N1 infection contamination have been accounted for; case-casualty rate is 53% (1-3). Most human contaminations with exceptionally pathogenic avian flu (HPAI) subtype H5N1 infection have happened following immediate or roundabout openness to tainted poultry in live-poultry markets (LPM) in agricultural nations (1-3). The principal risk factors

related with human diseases incorporate visiting a LPM or performing exercises with escalated contact with contaminated poultry, such as butchering, defeathering, or getting ready poultry for cooking (3,4).

Poultry-to-human avian flu (simulated intelligence) infection transmission can happen from 3 kinds of openness: fomite-contact transmission, incorporating contact with defiled surfaces; drop transmission, in which huge (>5 μm) particles contact an individual's conjunctiva or respiratory mucosa; and drop cores transmission (or spray transmission), in which an individual breathes in little (<5 μm) particles suspended in the air (5-8).

The LPM setting assumes a basic part in keeping up with, enhancing, and scattering artificial intelligence infections among poultry and from poultry to people (1,2,9), with backhanded proof of potential transmission through fomites, as upheld by the recognition of simulated intelligence infections in the climate (10-12), and airborne openness, upheld by the new segregation of flu And infections from air tested at LPMs in China (12). Moreover, suitable man-made intelligence infections can be distinguished in the air where live poultry are kept and handling exercises, for example, butchering and defeathering, are performed (12).

Aggregate epidemiologic and reconnaissance information propose that the butcher of tainted poultry is a significant general wellbeing concern. In our review, we verified that suitable airborne HPAI infection particles were created during reenacted handling of HPAI infection tainted poultry and that the airborne infection was communicated to infection guileless poultry and warm blooded creatures.

PREVENTION AND CONTROL

Biosecurity Measures

On the Ranch

Poultry makers ought to fortify biosecurity practices to forestall the presentation of HPAI into their herds. Coming up next are some strong biosecurity rehearses:

- Keep an "all-in, hard and fast" reasoning of the executives.

- Shield poultry runs from coming into contact with wild or transitory birds. Get poultry far from any wellspring of water that might have been tainted by wild birds.

- Grant just fundamental specialists and vehicles to enter the homestead.

- Give clean apparel and sanitization offices for workers.

- Completely perfect and sanitize gear and vehicles (counting tires and underside) entering and leaving the homestead.

- Try not to advance, or acquire gear or vehicles to/from different homesteads.

- Try not to visit other poultry ranches. In the event that you really do visit another homestead or live-bird market, change footwear and dress prior to working with your own herd.

- Try not to bring birds from butcher channels, particularly live-bird markets, back to the ranch.

At Live-Bird Markets (Domesticated animals Deal Offices)

To forestall a potential flare-up of HPAI, poultry makers and vendors should likewise utilize biosecurity safety measures at live-bird markets. Live-bird markets work in many significant urban areas.

Avian flu infections can be brought into these business sectors assuming they get tainted birds or sullied containers and trucks. When the infection is laid out on the lookout, the development of birds, containers, or trucks from a sullied market can spread the infection to different ranches and showcases.

Consequently, the accompanying defensive measures ought to be taken at live-bird markets to forestall the conceivable spread of illness:

Utilize plastic rather than wooden cases for simpler cleaning.

Keep scales and floors clean of fertilizer, feathers, and other trash.

Clean and sanitize all gear, cases, and vehicles prior to returning them to the homestead.

Continue approaching poultry separate from unsold birds, particularly assuming birds are from various parcels.

Clean and sanitize the commercial center after each day of offer.

Try not to return unsold birds to the homestead.

For more unambiguous data about biosecurity and cleaning and sterilization rehearses, contact your neighborhood USDA APHIS' Veterinary Administrations (Versus) office.

Vaccination Strategies

Vaccination Strategies include plans and strategies for regulating immunizations to a populace to accomplish explicit wellbeing results. These procedures can incorporate focusing on specific gatherings, similar to medical services laborers or high-risk people, sorting out mass inoculation crusades, guaranteeing fair conveyance, and carrying out instructive missions to advance immunization acknowledgment.

The effectiveness of vaccination strategies is simulated using mathematical modeling.
The information utilized were:

- Distributed writing (there were no limitations on distribution language or study area).
- Review information.
- Information on poultry populace in France, Italy and the Netherlands.
- Information on HPAI flare-ups in France, Italy and the Netherlands.

- Information on pre planned winnowing in France, Italy and the Netherlands.

What were the impediments/vulnerabilities?
Information on assurance viability and span of security of accessible immunizations against HPAI are non-fit and few; in this manner, the point by point depiction and correlation of these antibodies is absurd.

Hardly any antibodies are tried on poultry species other than chickens.

Field concentrates on the adequacy of immunization to stop infection transmission are scant.

What were the results and their suggestions?
Results

- Refreshed data was given on types and qualities of accessible antibodies against HPAI.
- There is just a single approved immunization against HPAI in chickens in the EU.
- Bits of knowledge were given on various immunization procedures to controlling HPAI in poultry, for example crisis defensive immunization in regions around a HPAI episode and preventive inoculation in regions and homesteads where the contamination is absent yet.
- Proposals were accommodated for future logical examinations on HPAI antibodies.

Suggestions

EFSA's logical counsel on HPAI antibodies and inoculation methodologies will illuminate EU Part State strategy creators and hazard directors about expected anticipation and control techniques for HPAI, hence empowering informed choices on HPAI counteraction and flare-up control. The exhortation from EFSA might direct future turn of events and utilization of immunizations against HPAI.

What are the key proposals?

Proposals for strategy producers and chance directors:

Preventive immunization is the ideal inoculation methodology to limit the quantity of flare-ups and term of plague and ought to be led in the most powerless and irresistible poultry species in high-risk transmission regions. Different organizations (for example sponsor immunizations) can be utilized to improve insurance.

In the event of an episode, crisis defensive immunization is suggested in a 3-km range of the flare-up in high-risk transmission regions.

Immunization viability ought to be checked for all inoculation procedures.
Immunization ought to supplement and not supplant other preventive and control measures, for example, contamination observing in birds, early discovery and biosecurity, and is suggested as a component of a coordinated infectious prevention approach.

Suggestions for the examination local area:

The logical assessment remembers proposals for future logical examinations for HPAI antibodies as far as the sorts of immunizations to create and for which bird species, the parts of the antibodies that ought to be explored and the kind of investigations that ought to be led.

ECONOMIC IMPACT

Agricultural Losses

Bird influenza, otherwise called avian flu, presents a critical danger to the worldwide poultry industry, prompting impressive rural misfortunes during episodes. The consequences of avian flu on farming are boundless, covering monetary misfortunes, disturbances in exchange, general wellbeing nerves, and the requirement for executing control systems.

1. Financial Setbacks: Avian flu flare-ups can have devastating monetary ramifications for poultry ranchers. This incorporates direct costs, for example, the deficiency of tainted birds because of mortality or winnowing to stop the infection's spread. In serious cases, whole rushes might expect willful extermination to contain the episode, bringing about significant monetary weights. Also, costs

related with executing biosecurity estimates like sanitization conventions and uplifted reconnaissance further add to the financial strain.

2. Trade Interruptions: Episodes of avian flu frequently trigger exchange limitations forced by bringing in countries to control the infection's spread by means of the worldwide development of poultry and related items. These embargoes can seriously influence nations intensely reliant upon poultry trades, prompting diminished market access and income slumps. Indeed, even areas unaffected by the episode might experience exchange boundaries because of worries about potential illness transmission.

3. Consumer Certainty Decline: Public confidence in the wellbeing of poultry items can wane during avian flu flare-ups, bringing about diminished customer interest. Apprehension about getting the infection from contaminated poultry items

can prompt decreased deals and utilization, fueling the monetary misfortunes for ranchers and the more extensive poultry industry. Reconstructing purchaser certainty frequently requires broad correspondence endeavors and confirmations in regards to sanitation measures.

4. Disruptions in Supply Chains: Avian flu flare-ups can disturb the whole poultry store network, from incubators and homesteads to handling offices and circulation organizations. Development limitations, quarantine measures, and eradication endeavors disturb the standard progression of labor and products, causing strategic obstacles and deficiencies in the store network. Handling plants might encounter brief terminations or decreased limit, influencing the opportune handling and dispersion of poultry items.

5. Environmental Consequences: The removal of tainted birds and polluted materials during avian flu flare-ups presents natural difficulties. Strategies like mass entombment, burning, or fertilizing the soil of corpses can bring about ecological repercussions, including soil and water defilement, as well as expected dangers to natural life and homegrown creatures. Legitimate removal methods should be utilized to alleviate the ecological effect and forestall further infection spread.

6. Long-Term Effects: Avian flu episodes can have getting through ramifications for impacted locales and the poultry business at large. Ranchers might confront critical monetary misfortunes, prompting ranch terminations, insolvency, or industry solidification. Besides, rehashed episodes can subvert buyer certainty and market steadiness, thwarting impacted locales' capacity to recover seriousness in the worldwide poultry market.

In synopsis, avian flu presents a diverse test to the horticultural area, causing significant monetary misfortunes, exchange disturbances, and general wellbeing concerns. Successful observation, biosecurity measures, and quick reaction capacities are critical for relieving the effect of avian flu episodes on poultry creation and defending the jobs of ranchers and industry partners.

Trade Disruptions

Avian flu, usually known as bird influenza, can fundamentally affect exchange, especially in the poultry business. Here is a top to bottom investigation of the exchange interruptions brought about by avian flu:

1. Market Closures: When a flare-up of avian flu happens, impacted nations frequently

close their homegrown and global business sectors to poultry items. This can incorporate live birds, poultry meat, eggs, and related items. Market terminations are executed to forestall the spread of the infection and safeguard general wellbeing.

2. Export Bans: Nations encountering avian flu episodes might force prohibitions on the commodity of poultry items. Regardless of whether a nation's own poultry industry isn't impacted, exchanging accomplices might force restrictions or limitations on imports from the impacted country because of worries about the spread of the infection. These commodity boycotts can have critical financial ramifications for the impacted country's poultry makers.

3. Loss of Customer Confidence: Avian flu flare-ups can prompt a deficiency of purchaser trust in poultry items, both locally and globally. Customers might become hesitant to buy poultry items because of a paranoid fear of getting the infection, regardless of whether the items are ok for utilization. This deficiency of certainty can additionally compound the monetary effect on the poultry business.

4. Supply Chain Disruptions: Avian flu episodes can upset the whole poultry inventory network, from creation and handling to dissemination and retail. Ranches might be compelled to winnow tainted birds, prompting a diminishing in supply. Handling plants might close down briefly to forestall the spread of the

infection. This can bring about deficiencies of poultry items and more exorbitant costs for customers.

5. Trade Negotiations: Avian flu episodes can likewise affect exchange discussions between nations. Exchanging accomplices might involve flare-ups as influence in dealings, requesting stricter measures to forestall the spread of the infection in return for lifting exchange limitations. This can prompt pressures among nations and defer the goal of exchange debates.

6. Long-Term Monetary Impact: The financial effect of avian flu episodes can stretch out past the quick emergency. Poultry makers might bring about huge monetary misfortunes because of

diminished request, winnowing of contaminated birds, and inflated costs related with biosecurity measures. The drawn out suitability of the poultry business in impacted nations might be raised doubt about, prompting rebuilding and solidification inside the business.

7. Global Exchange Stream Shifts: Avian flu flare-ups in significant poultry-creating nations can prompt changes in worldwide exchange streams. Bringing in nations might look for elective wellsprings of poultry items to supplant imports from impacted nations. This can set out open doors for poultry makers in different nations to grow their piece of the pie and increment sends out.

Generally speaking, avian flu flare-ups can have extensive ramifications for the worldwide poultry industry and global exchange. Successful reconnaissance, anticipation, and reaction measures are fundamental to relieve the effect of episodes and guarantee the proceeded with security and reasonability of the poultry exchange.

PANDEMIC PREPAREDNESS

Public Health Response

The public health response to avian influenza is multifaceted and involves various measures aimed at preventing the spread of the virus, protecting human health, and minimizing the impact of outbreaks. Here are some key aspects of the public health response to avian influenza:

1. Surveillance and Early Detection: Public health authorities closely monitor avian influenza outbreaks in both poultry and humans through surveillance systems. This includes monitoring wild bird populations, domestic poultry farms, and human cases of avian influenza. Early detection is crucial for implementing timely control measures and preventing further spread.

2. Risk Assessment and Communication: Public health agencies assess the risk posed by avian influenza outbreaks to human health and communicate relevant information to the public, healthcare providers, and other stakeholders. This includes providing guidance on preventive measures, symptoms to watch for, and actions to take in the event of suspected exposure.

3. Preventive Measures: Preventive measures are implemented to reduce the risk of human infection with avian influenza viruses. These measures may include:

- Promoting good hygiene practices, such as handwashing and respiratory etiquette.
- Advising people to avoid close contact with sick or dead birds.
- Recommending proper cooking of poultry products to kill any potential viruses.
- Providing personal protective equipment for individuals at high risk of exposure, such

as poultry workers and healthcare professionals.

4. Vaccination: In some cases, vaccination of poultry populations may be used as a preventive measure to reduce the spread of avian influenza viruses among birds. Vaccination can help reduce the likelihood of transmission to humans and prevent outbreaks in poultry farms.

5. Healthcare Preparedness: Public health agencies work to ensure that healthcare systems are prepared to respond to cases of avian influenza in humans. This includes:

- Training healthcare providers to recognize and manage suspected cases.
- Stockpiling antiviral medications for the treatment of human cases.
- Developing plans for surge capacity in healthcare facilities in the event of a large-scale outbreak.

6. International Collaboration: Avian influenza is a global health threat that requires international collaboration for effective control and response. Public health agencies, governments, and international organizations collaborate to share information, resources, and expertise to prevent the spread of the virus and mitigate its impact on human health.

7. Research and Development: Ongoing research is conducted to better understand avian influenza viruses, their transmission dynamics, and potential interventions. This includes vaccine development, antiviral drug research, and studies on the ecology of avian influenza viruses in both bird and human populations.

By implementing comprehensive public health measures, countries can mitigate the risk of avian influenza outbreaks, protect human health, and maintain confidence in poultry products and the food supply. Early detection, effective communication, and coordinated response efforts are essential components of a successful public health response to avian influenza.

Risk Mitigation Strategies

Risk relief systems for avian flu include a mix of measures pointed toward forestalling the spread of the infection among poultry and people, diminishing the probability of flare-ups, and limiting the effect of any potential episodes that do happen. Here is a broad gander at some key gamble moderation techniques:

1. Biosecurity Measures: Executing severe biosecurity estimates on poultry ranches is fundamental for forestalling the presentation and spread of avian flu infections. This incorporates controlling admittance to ranches, cleaning vehicles and hardware, forestalling contact between wild birds and poultry, and keeping up with great cleanliness rehearses among ranch laborers.

2. Surveillance and Early Detection: Early discovery of avian flu episodes is basic for executing ideal control measures. Reconnaissance frameworks ought to be set up to screen poultry populaces for indications of infection, as well as wild bird populaces for the presence of avian flu infections. Fast symptomatic tests can assist with distinguishing tainted birds rapidly, taking into account brief activity to contain the infection.

3. Vaccination Programs: Immunization of poultry populaces can assist with lessening the spread of avian flu infections and relieve the effect of episodes. Immunizations are accessible for specific types of avian flu and are utilized in locales where the infection is endemic or where there is a high gamble of transmission. Immunization procedures ought to be customized to the particular attributes of the infection and the neighborhood poultry populace.

4. Quarantine and Development Controls: Executing quarantine measures and development controls can assist with forestalling the spread of avian flu between poultry homesteads and areas. Tainted ranches ought to be separated, and development of birds, individuals, and gear ought to be confined to forestall further transmission. Powerful coordination between government organizations and partners is fundamental for implementing quarantine gauges and controlling the development of poultry and poultry items.

5. Risk Correspondence and Public Awareness: Public mindfulness missions can assist with instructing poultry makers, laborers, and the overall population about avian flu dangers and preventive measures. Clear and opportune correspondence of data about episodes, biosecurity practices, and inoculation projects can assist advance

consistence with risk alleviation gauges and lessen the spread of the infection.

6. International Cooperation: Avian flu is a transboundary danger that requires collaboration between nations to successfully oversee and control. Global associations like the World Wellbeing Association (WHO), the World Association for Creature Wellbeing (OIE), and the Food and Farming Association (FAO) work with coordinated effort and data dividing among nations. Joint observation endeavors, limit building drives, and reaction coordination instruments assist with reinforcing worldwide readiness and reaction to avian flu.

7. Research and Innovation: Proceeded with exploration and advancement are fundamental for growing new apparatuses and procedures for avian flu risk alleviation. This remembers research for infection transmission elements, immunization

advancement, symptomatic methods, and elective control measures. Interest in innovative work can prompt more powerful mediations for forestalling and controlling avian flu episodes later on.

By carrying out a far reaching way to deal with risk relief that consolidates these systems, nations can decrease the probability of avian flu episodes, safeguard poultry and human wellbeing, and shield food security and exchange. Powerful gamble relief requires coordinated effort between government organizations, the poultry business, general wellbeing specialists, and global accomplices to address the intricate difficulties presented by avian flu.

FUTURE RESEARCH DIRECTIONS

Antiviral Development

The improvement of antiviral medications for avian flu is a basic part of endeavors to battle the spread of the infection and decrease its effect on human and creature wellbeing. Antiviral medications are intended to hinder the replication of flu infections, including those that taint birds and can possibly communicate to people. Here is a broad investigation of antiviral advancement for avian flu:

1. Targeting Viral Replication: Antiviral medications for avian flu commonly target key proteins or cycles engaged with the replication of the infection. One normal objective is the viral compound neuraminidase, which assumes a critical part in the arrival of recently shaped infection particles from tainted cells.

Neuraminidase inhibitors, for example, oseltamivir (Tamiflu) and zanamivir (Relenza), are broadly involved antiviral medications for both occasional and avian flu.

2. Broad-Range Antivirals: Scientists are additionally investigating the advancement of expansive range antiviral medications that can restrain numerous types of flu infections, incorporating those with pandemic potential. These medications target rationed districts of the infection that are less inclined to transform and foster obstruction. Models incorporate favipiravir and baloxavir marboxil, which have shown viability against different flu strains in preclinical and clinical examinations.

3. Resistance Observing and Management: One test in the turn of events and utilization of antiviral medications for avian flu is the potential for the development of medication safe strains. Nonstop observing of circling

infections for opposition transformations is fundamental for early location of obstruction and illuminating treatment rules. Methodologies for overseeing opposition incorporate blend treatment, which includes utilizing numerous antiviral medications with various systems of activity to lessen the gamble of obstruction advancement.

4. New Medication Discovery: Exploration endeavors are continuous to find novel antiviral mixtures with further developed adequacy, wellbeing, and opposition profiles. High-throughput screening of synthetic libraries, structure-based drug plan, and computational demonstrating are utilized to distinguish promising medication applicants. Regular items, engineered compounds, and reused drugs are being researched for their true capacity as antiviral specialists against avian flu.

5. Animal Models and Clinical Trials: Creature models of avian flu contamination, like mice, ferrets, and non-human primates, are utilized to assess the viability and security of antiviral medications in preclinical examinations. Clinical preliminaries in people are then led to evaluate the wellbeing, pharmacokinetics, and antiviral action of applicant drugs. These preliminaries might include solid workers or people tainted with avian flu under controlled conditions.

6. Regulatory Endorsement and Access: Antiviral medications for avian flu should go through thorough administrative survey and endorsement processes before they can be made accessible for clinical use. Administrative organizations, like the U.S. Food and Medication Organization (FDA) and the European Meds Organization (EMA), assess information from preclinical and clinical examinations to decide the wellbeing and adequacy of new medications.

Once supported, endeavors are made to guarantee admittance to these medications in districts where avian flu is endemic or episodes happen.

7. Global Cooperation and Partnership: Joint effort between legislatures, scholarly establishments, drug organizations, and global associations is fundamental for propelling antiviral advancement for avian flu. Drives like the Worldwide Drive on Sharing Avian Flu Information (GISAID) work with information dividing and cooperation among specialists around the world. Public-private organizations, like the Alliance for Pandemic Readiness Advancements (CEPI), give financing and backing to innovative work of antibodies and antiviral medications for arising irresistible sicknesses, including avian flu.

By putting resources into examination, advancement, and coordinated effort, progress keeps on being made in the improvement of antiviral medications for avian flu. These medications assume a pivotal part in the counteraction, treatment, and control of avian flu flare-ups, assisting with defending general wellbeing and moderate the effect of the infection on worldwide wellbeing security.

Surveillance Enhancements

Surveillance enhancements for avian influenza are crucial for early detection, monitoring, and control of the virus in both poultry and human populations. Advances in surveillance technology, data collection methods, and data analysis techniques have improved our ability to detect and respond to avian influenza outbreaks more rapidly and effectively. Here's an extensive exploration of surveillance enhancements for avian influenza:

1. Remote Sensing and Geographic Information Systems (GIS): Remote sensing technologies, such as satellite imagery and

aerial photography, can be used to monitor environmental factors that influence the spread of avian influenza, such as bird migration patterns, water sources, and land use changes. Geographic Information Systems (GIS) allow for the integration and analysis of spatial data, helping to identify high-risk areas and target surveillance efforts more effectively.

2. Real-Time Polymerase Chain Reaction (PCR) Testing: Real-time PCR testing allows for rapid and accurate detection of avian influenza viruses in poultry and environmental samples. This molecular diagnostic technique amplifies and detects viral nucleic acids in real time, providing results within hours. Real-time PCR testing is widely used in surveillance programs to screen large numbers of samples quickly and identify infected flocks or regions.

3. Next-Generation Sequencing (NGS): Next-generation sequencing technologies

have revolutionized the field of molecular epidemiology by enabling high-throughput sequencing of viral genomes. NGS allows for the rapid and comprehensive analysis of avian influenza viruses, including their genetic diversity, evolution, and transmission dynamics. This information is essential for tracking the spread of the virus, identifying new strains, and assessing their potential threat to human and animal health.

4. Syndromic Surveillance: Syndromic surveillance involves monitoring specific clinical signs or symptoms in humans or animals that may indicate the presence of avian influenza. In humans, syndromic surveillance systems can track influenza-like illness (ILI) symptoms reported by healthcare providers or individuals in real time. In animals, surveillance systems may monitor for signs of respiratory disease or unusual mortality events in poultry flocks. Early detection of syndromic signals can

trigger rapid response actions to investigate and control potential outbreaks.

5. One Health Surveillance: One Health surveillance approaches integrate data from multiple sectors, including human health, animal health, and environmental health, to better understand and address the complex interactions between humans, animals, and their shared environments. One Health surveillance efforts for avian influenza involve collaboration between public health agencies, veterinary authorities, environmental agencies, and other stakeholders to monitor and mitigate the risk of zoonotic transmission.

6. Surveillance Networks and Information Sharing: Surveillance networks facilitate the sharing of data, information, and resources between countries and regions to enhance global surveillance and response to avian influenza. International organizations such as the World Health Organization (WHO),

the World Organisation for Animal Health (OIE), and the Food and Agriculture Organization (FAO) coordinate surveillance activities, provide technical assistance, and promote data sharing through platforms like the Global Early Warning System (GLEWS) and the Global Influenza Surveillance and Response System (GISRS).

7. Capacity Building and Training: Capacity building initiatives aim to strengthen surveillance capabilities at the local, national, and regional levels through training, infrastructure development, and resource mobilization. Training programs for laboratory technicians, epidemiologists, veterinarians, and other surveillance personnel enhance their skills in sample collection, testing, data analysis, and outbreak response. Investment in laboratory infrastructure, equipment, and diagnostic reagents is essential for building sustainable surveillance systems in resource-limited settings.

By leveraging advances in surveillance technology, data analysis, and interdisciplinary collaboration, surveillance enhancements for avian influenza contribute to more effective prevention, detection, and control of the virus, ultimately reducing the risk of outbreaks and protecting public health.

CONCLUSION

In the book discussing avian influenza, readers are taken on an exploration of the intricate realm of one of humanity's most captivating yet enigmatic viruses. Through its pages, a trove of intriguing insights into the biology, ecology, and epidemiology of avian influenza is unveiled, revealing the intricate web of interactions that govern its emergence, transmission, and impact on both animal and human populations.

Starting from its origins within wild bird populations, avian influenza's occasional incursions into domestic poultry and, more rarely, into humans are vividly portrayed, highlighting the ever-present threat that looms on the fringes of our interconnected world. Readers are immersed in the exploration of viral evolution, genetic variability, and the intricate dance between hosts and pathogens, shedding light on the mechanisms underlying the virus's ability to persist, evolve, and sporadically spark devastating outbreaks.

Throughout the narrative, readers encounter the unsung heroes of the story: the dedicated scientists, veterinarians, healthcare workers, and policymakers who labor tirelessly to unravel the virus's mysteries, pioneer innovative surveillance techniques, and implement effective control measures. Their relentless efforts underscore the paramount importance of interdisciplinary collaboration, data exchange, and global solidarity in confronting the multifaceted challenges posed by avian influenza.

However, interspersed among tales of scientific discovery and public health interventions, the book also lays bare the profound socio-economic ramifications of avian influenza, from the crippling losses suffered by poultry farmers to the disruptions in international trade and food security. These narratives serve as poignant reminders of the wide-ranging repercussions of infectious disease outbreaks and underscore the urgent imperative for preparedness and resilience in the face of emerging threats.

As readers reach the conclusion of the book, they are left with a profound appreciation for the intricacies and resilience of life on our planet. Avian influenza emerges not merely as a biological phenomenon but as a reflection of the delicate equilibrium between humans, animals, and the environment—a testament to our interconnectedness and shared obligation to safeguard the health and well-being of all living beings.

Ultimately, the book on avian influenza imparts not only a deeper comprehension of the virus but also instills a sense of hope and determination. Armed with knowledge, insight, and a commitment to collective action, we can confront the challenges posed by avian influenza and steer towards a future that is safer, healthier, and more resilient for all.

www.ingramcontent.com/pod-product-compliance
Lightning Source LLC
Chambersburg PA
CBHW070122230526
45472CB00004B/1374
* 9 7 9 8 3 2 7 7 8 0 8 1 1 *